A Royal Priesthood

Nutritional Care of the
Holy Temple of God

By

Deborah Gilbreath

A Royal Priesthood

1 Peter 2:9

But ye are a chosen generation,
a **royal priest**hood,
an holy nation, a peculiar people;
that ye should shew forth the praises
of him who hath called you out of
darkness into his marvelous light;

We are all born with a human body that requires nutritional intake in order to function and grow properly. Infants cry to let their mother know that they are hungry and need to eat. Older people recognize a growling stomach as a sign that it is time to feed their body some food and stop the growling. Human digestion starts in the mouth and the mouth waters at the thought of good food or at the sight and smell of good food. This is part of the process that begins to break down the food that we eat as we chew it up.

We develop attitudes about eating starting with the baby's breastfeeding experience or bottle feeding experience. Those who receive good bonding with their parent can have security and confidence that their nutritional needs will be met and that they can trust the parent to supply their needs. Some parents are nervous and anxious about the feeding and convey this emotion to the baby thus generating mealtime anxiety.

Some parents tend to overfeed the baby stretching the stomach too much and too often leading to an abnormal need for excess food. Thus in older children, food is often used as a reward for desired behavior and treats are withheld as a punishment for undesired behavior. Advertisers highlight the joy of consuming their colorful and flavorful foods on television, in magazines and on billboards. All these cues to eat stimulate the appetite and cause us to want to eat for other reasons that the actual hunger response our body gives us when we need food.

Food is often used to comfort people when they are sad or feeling depressed. Friends or loved ones may linger and share loving conversation over blueberry muffins or banana bread. Perhaps we are given ice cream after having our feelings hurt by the other children. These situations help to reinforce that food is good for healing the emotions and sets us up to 'eat at' our emotions, rather than to learn to feel our feelings and process our emotions in more healthy ways.

In some cases meals are not provided on a regular schedule or the amounts of food may be sparse and not enough to satisfy the appetite.can generate anxiety about meals and anger and rage associated with hunger. Feelings of having been deprived may lead to overeating in later years when more food, or better food, is available.

Social events often center around a meal and, in America at Christmas and Thanksgiving, may be a time when people eat holiday foods until they are uncomfortably full. These times are often associate with intense emotions of love, or stress, depending on the family interpersonal and emotional dynamics. Seasonal treats abound in all the magazines and on the internet to help us to get ready and celebrate the holiday, the season or the social event. To fail to indulge is to be left out of the festivities, or so it seems.

These are the voices of the word and the way that the

world trains us to obey our flesh when our flesh indicates that it would prefer to eat and what it would prefer to eat.

Later on in life, many of us tend to put on extra pounds with this eating pattern that develops in childhood. Sedentary lifestyle and eating when we are hungry add weight faster than we can burn it off and obesity is the result.

Now come that many different drastic dieting methods that may take off a few pounds, or even quite a few pounds, for a short time. The sad outcome is that many of us suffer from a yo yo effect and gain back all the weight that we lost and then some, so that we end up weighing more than when we started on the diet.

Then there are childhood traumas such as abusive situations that may or may not include eating and food. Many people continue to suffer from the trauma of childhood abuse and this is exhibited in starving themselves or overeating to the point of binging, using diuretics and laxatives to lose weight and making oneself to throw up, called purging. Some people are exercise fanatics due to an unrealistic body image or unrealistic goals for their age or body type.

Normal nutritional values for a healthy dietary intake are 45% to 65% Carbohydrates, 10% to 35% Protein and 20% to 35% fats according to the Mayo Clinic. Fiber is important and comes from fruits and vegetables. Women need 22 to 28 grams of fiber per day and men need 28 to 34 grams per day.

Many diets that are being promoted eliminate some of these essential and necessary elements or drastically alter the amount being eaten. These are what I call *heroic* or drastic measures.

When a person accepts Lord Jesus Christ as the Savior, confesses that they are a sinner and need to be saved, believes that God raised Jesus from the dead, and trusts Jesus as Lord over their life they receive Eternal

Life in Jesus Christ. At this time Jesus sends the Holy Spirit to dwell in that person as a companion, teacher, helper, and to signify to God that the person belongs to Christ. This is when the human body become a Temple of the Living God, or a Holy Temple. Many of us have already developed poor eating and nutrition habits by the time this event occurs in our lives. Thus we are not in a position to properly care for and beautify our body Temple for the glory of God and the vitality of the Holy Spirit.

Our appetites have been causing us trouble since the Fall in the Garden of Eden when Satan whetted Eve's appetite for fruit that she did not need to be hungry for because all of her nutritional needs had been graciously and lovingly provided for by God Himself. Eve failed to rely on God whole-heartedly and to stand firm in her relationship with God, she was distracted by the allure of something that she should not eat.

This leads us to the topic of refined sugar. Refined sugar is very addicting to many people and it yields metabolic highs and crashing lows with resultant craving for more sugar. This throws our digestive system off balance from the healthy normal and creates a roller coaster effect that can affect our emotions and peace of mind. The Mayo clinic recommends that we get no more than 100 calories per day of refined sugar for women and 150 for men. I have found that removing refined sugar from the diet altogether on most days is the best policy in order to prevent highs and lows and feelings of craving. Therefore, refined sugars defile the Holy Temple of God when careful moderation is not practiced.

1 Corinthians 3:17

If any man **defile the temple** of God, him shall God destroy; for **the temple** of God is holy, which **temple** ye are.

We do not have to go far to realize that refined sugars are defiling and destroying the body Temple of many people all over the world, as evidenced by obesity and Diabetes in the population. Historically, advertisers have been oblivious to this dilemma and have simply sought to ring up sales of sugary products by hard selling them in commercials and in playing on our impulse buying habits by placing them all at the cash register area to make us think that we are hungry now. Such is the way of the world and it was the way of the world when Daniel was captive in Babylon and the king ordered the Babylonian diet for Daniel and his fellows.

Daniel 1:8

But **Daniel purposed in his heart** that he would not defile himself with the portion of the king's meat, nor with the wine which he drank: therefore he requested of the prince of the eunuchs that he might not defile himself.

It will take most of us a concentrated effort and the help of Lord Jesus Christ in order to avoid defiling ourselves with excessive refined sugars. The first thing that many of us must do is to begin

to record what we are eating each day on paper, just to get an honest appraisal of where we are at the starting point; without making any changes in dietary habits. Even this is uncomfortable and requires great faith and devotion to develop a discipline for doing it.

As I looked over my daily dietary intake sheet I asked myself "Would I feed a child that I was caring for this way?" The answer in my case was "No!" I found that I was eating at erratic times during the day and taking in quite a bit of refined sugars. I decided to write "**Child of God**" at the top of my dietary intake record so that I remembered to be responsible in the care of the Holy Temple of God that is my body. A responsible and loving way to feed a child would be 3 balanced meals per day with 1 or 2 healthy snacks. This would be our first goal in properly fueling the Holy Temple of God with adequate nutrition.

It usually takes about 72 hours to withdraw from many substances and cutting out the refined sugar made me uncomfortable, jittery, and irritable and gave me a headache for about 3 days, but then I got used to it. Fruit tasted sweeter after I got off refined sugars. I love to eat fruit flavored yogurt with an artificial sweetener in it. After about 2 weeks I no longer missed or thought about refined sugars. I had made up my mind not to be defiled by them anymore by excessive and regular intake. After this has become a firmly established habit one can

start with. I have chosen to walk 30 minutes per day 3 times a week as my regular exercise program. This is moderate and it boosts the metabolism and strengthens my bones and muscles.

An added benefit of walking is that one can wear headphones and listen to Christian praise and worship music while walking and this turns exercise time into a time of prayer, meditation and talking to Jesus while enjoying lively music. I really come alive during these sessions and feel exhilarated and energized after my walk. I am filled with hope for the future and love for God and occasionally have a cookie or an ice cream using compassionate moderation as the guiding principle. Putting the care of my body Temple under the direct control and management of Jesus Christ means that I do not have to obsess or be compulsive in eating patterns or dietary control.

Each day I pray and dedicate my life to Jesus Christ and I ask Him to grant me physical fitness, appetite suppression and control, weight loss, and the beauty of the Lord in my body, soul and spirit. This means that I need to add exercise to my program of care for the Holy

Temple of God. Again, I do not want to be obsessive or focus on my weight. We are looking for compassionate moderation and recovery from sluggishness. We are not training for the Olympics or fixing ideals on a particular weight. A joyous spirit and a smooth-running healthy Temple are worthy goals to man after all that praise and worship music.

Water is very important to create a good metabolic environment in the Holy Temple of God, which is your body. Mayo clinic recommends 8 eight ounce glasses of water a day in one article. This purifies and flushes the body Temple and keeps it running efficiently.

After monitoring the diet for 2 to 4 weeks and simply trying to eat 3 balanced meals a day with 1 or 2 snacks we will want to begin to record the daily caloric intake that we are eating. Compare this with the maintenance level of calories needed for your age, height and activity level. There are many internet sites that calculate daily caloric needs and many of them come up with vastly different numbers. I took the figure which seemed to be in the center of the two extremes. In my case, I weighed 195 pounds and I wanted to keep from gaining weight so I figured out that my daily maintenance calories would be about 2032 per day.

My inner nature rebelled against all the light being shed on my eating habits and I was quite nervous for a couple of weeks even though I knew that I was getting enough food for my body and that I was being fed on regular intervals in a healthy way. After years of darkness in the area of my awareness of my nutritional intake and just eating what I wanted, when I was hungry this seemed like a massive intrusion into my own privacy and rights. Now, I realized that I was touching on the emotional aspects of my eating habits and I chose to work a 12 Step program for recovery at a local church called 'Celebrate Recovery'. This has helped a lot with eradicating the emotional cues to eat that once drove my appetites and behaviors.

After about 5 weeks of maintenance calories every day, I decided to go down to 1900 calories per day. Going down on calories in small increments every 4 to 6 weeks is an easier way to adjust myself to regulating my dietary intake. This generated a feeling of hunger in me every now and then which I treated with Garcenia Cambrogia tablets purchased at the local drug store. I take 1600 mg in the morning and late afternoon and this prevents me from feeling hungry during the day.

In order to maintain a good balance of nutrition during the day and to feel full in the evening so that I could sleep better I divided my daily calories by 7 and planned to take 2/7 in the morning hours, 2/7 in the afternoon hours and 3/7 at the evening meal.

For a 1900 calorie a day diet this was 543 in the morning, 543 in the afternoon and 814 at night. Of course this is not iron clad or written in stone and I frequently take in fewer calories in the morning and a few more a supper time. For me the main thing is to be a joyous Temple of the Living God most of the time and not to be suffering and obsessing about food, eating, diet or exercise. Focusing on those things is all about focusing on me. As a Christian, I want to focus more on my relationship with Jesus Christ and my Christian walk than I do on myself.

The best way to avoid thinking about myself is to think about being of service to the people that God has placed in my life for me to minister to, starting at home. Caring for and about the needs of others takes the focus off myself and lessens the incidence of perceived hunger that is really caused by boredom, discontent or emotional disturbances.

All aspects of the Holy Temple of God should be properly fueled and nourished. Keeping a daily record of my dietary intake for the "**Child of God**" that I am gives me a chance to pray over the day's intake and to confess to God any shortcomings and to ask for His help with the next day's efforts. This daily confession is an important part of my spiritual life and relationship with God. Also, the daily intake record serves as a fuel gauge for how I am fueling the Temple of God. Am I flooding the engine at times with excessive food intake? Am I running out of gas at certain times? Am I filling the tank on a regular basis with moderate meals at appropriate times? If I know that I am doing all these things then I know that the idea that I want to eat when it is not a meal or snack time is coming from emotional and psychological causes and I can turn it over to God in prayer and ask Him to take the craving away from me and direct my attention to what he would have me to do.

It is important to feed the Spirit on the Word of God every day and to nourish my Soul with prayer and meditation with God

on a daily basis. I truly love Psalm 119 for the purpose of celebrating the importance of learning about God's Word and meditating on that Word daily. There are unlimited benefits to studying the Holy Bible for improving our lives and the lives of those that we are associated with. Psalm 119 is written with the letter of the Hebrew alphabet at the top of each section for all the letters. This makes it the longest Psalm, but it is chocked full of good encouragement and teaching and should be read and carefully considered by those who want to have an effective spiritual boost to their fitness and beauty program. Remembering that God is in charge of my life and in charge of my Holy Temple of God, which is my body, keeps everything in right and true perspective. Remembering the price that Jesus paid to save me from my despair and sin helps me to want to care for the dwelling of the Holy Spirit in a more loving and responsible way.

1 Corinthians 6:20

For ye are bought with a price: therefore glorify God in your body, and in your spirit, which are God's.

All Christians belong to God and each one is a Temple for the Living God. Within the Body of Christ we are all members of one another and when one suffers we all suffer. Caring for my body Temple is a loving way that I can be a good influence on the Body of Christ by spiritual means. My health and beauty increases the health and beauty of the body and affects others. I want to do all that I can to strengthen and promote the Body of Christ here on the earth and to see His will done in this world. Caring for a Holy Temple of God is a stewardship trust that lasts for the rest of my life. This means that I will be monitoring my dietary intake on paper for the rest of my life as a daily inventory. It means that I will be exercising moderately each week on a regular basis and that I will be making healthy dietary choices.

Planning and recording of dietary intake takes the fight or flight adrenalin response of fear and rage out of my dietary practices. When we take anything away we should add something positive in

its place. Planning and recording adds regularity, stability, faithfulness, love and dependability into my dietary practices. I can know that I am caring for the **"Child of God"** that I am in a responsible way and being a good steward of my Master's resources. This takes the stress out of the question "What am I going to eat?"

A little planning goes a long way to prevent binges and famines.

Just as God removed all the giant number of troops from Gideon when he was going to battle against the Midianites, we remove all the drastic, stringent and heroic diet and weight loss strategies and instead adapt a completely new lifestyle. Each day I pray that God will give me a completely new attitude and a new strength and resolve about eating, diet, nutrition and body image. I stay off the scale completely. There is no magic number of happiness in the world of weight control. I try to stay at a particular calorie level for 5 to 6 weeks before thinking about going down to a lower level. I am totally disregarding extreme fat burning weight loss calorie recommendations. I put the weight on slowly and it can come off slowly as well. Nothing is worth losing my joy and peace over in my relationship with the Lord.

I am blessed in the dietary maintenance of my body Temple with the unrushed grace of God and no deadlines. My affirmation is "The Lord refurnishes, restores and beautifies my body Temple." Jesus is able to completely rebuild me from the inside out and to change all aspects of my life for the better as I invite Him to take control more and more of every detail of my life. May God richly bless you in the nutritional care of your body Temple.

Deborah Gilbreath is a second year seminary student in Dallas, Texas who is studying for a Master of Divinity degree. She is a former member of TOPS weight loss club as well as Overeaters Anonymous. She has taken two nutrition for science majors courses at college and has a lifetime of experience with unhealthy weight loss strategies prior to turning her life over to Jesus Christ as Lord and Savior over her life. Christ promises us a new life and a new outlook and attitude as well as new habits of nutrition are all part of that new life. She is the 12 Step mentor of women who want to change their lives through the power of Jesus Christ.